# The Ultimate Sweet Chaffle Cookbook

*Simple Recipes for your Sweet Moments*

*Imogene Cook*

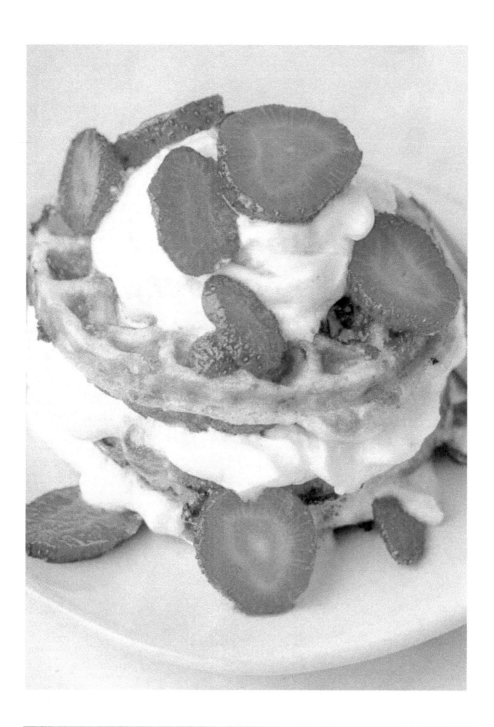

# TABLE OF CONTENTS

# How to Make Chaffles?

## Equipment and Ingredients Discussed

Making chaffles requires five simple steps and nothing more than a waffle maker for flat chaffles and a waffle bowl maker for chaffle bowls.

To make chaffles, you will need two necessary ingredients —eggs and cheese. My preferred cheeses are cheddar cheese or mozzarella cheese. These melt quickly, making them the go-to for most recipes. Meanwhile, always ensure that your cheeses are finely grated or thinly sliced for use.

Now, to make a standard chaffle:

First, preheat your waffle maker until adequately hot.

Meanwhile, in a bowl, mix the egg with cheese on hand until well combined.

Open the iron, pour in a quarter or half of the mixture, and close.

Cook the chaffle for 5 to 7 minutes or until it is crispy.

Transfer the chaffle to a plate and allow cooling before serving.

## 11 Tips to Make Chaffles

My surefire ways to turn out the crispiest of chaffles:

**Preheat Well:** Yes! It sounds obvious to preheat the waffle iron before usage. However, preheating the iron moderately

will not get your chaffles as crispy as you will like. The best way to preheat before cooking is to ensure that the iron is very hot.

**Not-So-Cheesy:** Will you prefer to have your chaffles less cheesy? Then use mozzarella cheese.

**Not-So Eggy**: If you aren't comfortable with the smell of eggs in your chaffles, try using egg whites instead of egg yolks or whole eggs.

**To Shred or to Slice:** Many recipes call for shredded cheese when making chaffles, but I find sliced cheeses to offer crispier pieces. While I stick with mostly shredded cheese for convenience's sake, be at ease to use sliced cheese in the same quantity. When using sliced cheeses, arrange two to four pieces in the waffle iron, top with the beaten eggs, and some slices of the cheese. Cover and cook until crispy.

**Shallower Irons:** For better crisps on your chaffles, use shallower waffle irons as they cook easier and faster.

**Layering:** Don't fill up the waffle iron with too much batter. Work between a quarter and a half cup of total ingredients per batch for correctly done chaffles.

**Patience:** It is a virtue even when making chaffles. For the best results, allow the chaffles to sit in the iron for 5 to 7 minutes before serving.

**No Peeking:** 7 minutes isn't too much of a time to wait for the outcome of your chaffles, in my opinion.

Opening the iron and checking on the chaffle before

it is done stands you a worse chance of ruining it.

**Crispy Cooling:** For better crisp, I find that allowing the chaffles to cool further after they are transferred to a plate aids a lot.

**Easy Cleaning:** For the best cleanup, wet a paper towel and wipe the inner parts of the iron clean while still warm. Kindly note that the iron should be warm but not hot!

**Brush It:** Also, use a clean toothbrush to clean between the iron's teeth for a thorough cleanup. You may also use a dry, rough sponge to clean the iron while it is still warm.

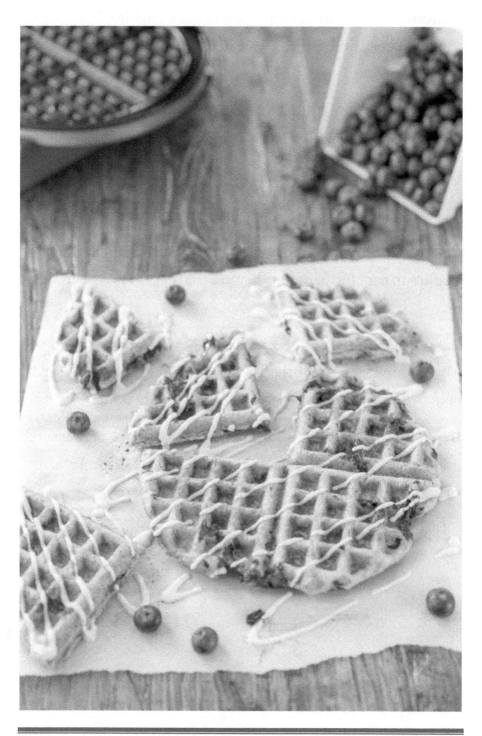

# Basic Keto Chaffles

Preparation time: 5 minutes

Cooking Time: 5 Minutes

Servings: 2

## Ingredients:

- 1 egg
- ½ cup shredded Cheddar cheese

## Directions:

1. Turn on waffle maker to heat and oil it with cooking spray.
2. Whisk egg in a bowl until well beaten.
3. Add cheese to the egg and stir well to combine.
4. Pour ½ batter into the waffle maker and close the top. Cook for 3-5 minutes.
5. Transfer chaffle to a plate and set aside for 2-3 minutes to crisp up.
6. Repeat for remaining batter.

## Nutrition: Carbs:

1 g ; Fat: 12 g ;Protein: 9 g ;Calories: 150

# Red Velvet Chaffles

Preparation time: 5 minutes

Cooking Time: 8 Minutes

Servings: 2

## Ingredients:

- 2 tablespoons cacao powder
- 2 tablespoons erythritol
- 1 organic egg, beaten
- 2 drops super red food coloring
- ¼ teaspoon organic baking powder
- 1 tablespoon heavy whipping cream

## Directions:

1. Preheat a mini waffle iron and then grease it.
2. In a medium bowl, put all ingredients and with a fork, mix until well combined.
3. Place half of the mixture into preheated waffle iron and cook for about 4 minutes.
4. Repeat with the remaining mixture.

5. Serve warm.

6.

## Nutrition:

Calories 70 Net Carbs 1.7 g Total Fat g Saturated Fat 3 g Cholesterol 92 mg Sodium 34 mg Total Carbs 3.2 g Fiber 1.5 g Sugar 0.2 g Protein 3.9 g

# Mayonnaise Chaffles

Preparation time: 5 minutes

Cooking Time: 10 Minutes

Servings: 3

## Ingredients:

- 1 large organic egg, beaten
- 1 tablespoon mayonnaise
- 2 tablespoons almond flour
- 1/8 teaspoon organic baking powder
- 1 teaspoon water
- 2–4 drops liquid stevia

## Directions:

1. Preheat a mini waffle iron and then grease it.
2. In a medium bowl, put all ingredients and with a fork, mix until well combined. Place half of the mixture into preheated waffle iron and cook for about 4–5 minutes.
3. Repeat with the remaining mixture.
4. Serve warm.

**Nutrition:**

Calories 110 Net Carbs 2.6 g Total Fat 8.7 g Saturated Fat 1.4 g Cholesterol 9mg Sodium 88 g Total Carbs 3.4 g Fiber 0.8 g Sugar 0.9 g Protein 3.2 g

# Chocolate Peanut Butter Chaffle

Preparation time: 5 minutes

Cooking Time: 10 Minutes

Servings: 2

## Ingredients:

- ½ cup shredded mozzarella cheese
- 1 Tbsp cocoa powder
- 2 Tbsp powdered sweetener
- 2 Tbsp peanut butter
- ½ tsp vanilla
- 1 egg
- 2 Tbsp crushed peanuts
- 2 Tbsp whipped cream
- ¼ cup sugar-free chocolate syrup

## Directions:

1. Combine mozzarella, egg, vanilla, peanut butter, cocoa powder, and sweetener in a bowl.
2. Add in peanuts and mix well.

3. Turn on waffle maker and oil it with cooking spray.

4. Pour one half of the batter into waffle maker and cook for minutes, then transfer to a plate.

5. Top with whipped cream, peanuts, and sugar-free chocolate syrup.

**Nutrition:**

Carbs: g ; Fat: 17 g ;Protein: 15 g ;Calories: 236

# Lemon Curd Chaffles

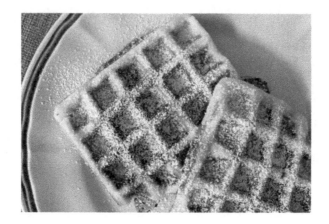

Preparation time: 5 minute

Servings: 1

Cooking Time: 5 Minutes

**Ingredients:**

- 3 large eggs
- 4 oz cream cheese, softened
- 1 Tbsp low carb sweetener
- 1 tsp vanilla extract
- ¾ cup mozzarella cheese, shredded
- 3 Tbsp coconut flour
- 1 tsp baking powder

- ⅓ tsp salt

## For the lemon curd:

- ½-1 cup water
- 5 egg yolks
- ½ cup lemon juice
- ½ cup powdered sweetener
- 2 Tbsp fresh lemon zest
- 1 tsp vanilla extract
- Pinch of salt
- 8 Tbsp cold butter, cubed

## Directions:

1. Pour water into a saucepan and heat over medium until it reaches a soft boil. Start with ½ cup and add more if needed.
2. Whisk yolks, lemon juice, lemon zest, powdered sweetener, vanilla, and salt in a medium heat-proof bowl. Leave to set for 5-6 minutes.
3. Place bowl onto saucepan and heat. The bowl shouldn't be touching water.
4. Whisk mixture for 8-10 minutes, or until it begins to thicken.
5. Add butter cubes and whisk for 7 minutes, until it thickens.

6. When it lightly coats the back of a spoon, remove from heat.

7. Refrigerate until cool, allowing it to continue thickening.

8. Turn on waffle maker to heat and oil it with cooking spray.

9. Add baking powder, coconut flour, and salt in a small bowl. Mix well and set aside.

10. Add eggs, cream cheese, sweetener, and vanilla in a separate bowl. Using a hand beater, beat until frothy.

11. Add mozzarella to egg mixture and beat again.

12. Add dry ingredients and mix until well-combined.

13. Add batter to waffle maker and cook for 3-4

14. minutes.

15. Transfer to a plate and top with lemon curd before serving.

**Nutrition:**

Carbs: 6 g; Fat: 24 g ;Protein: g Calories –302

# Walnut Pumpkin Chaffles

Preparation time: 5 minutes

Cooking Time: 10 Minutes

Servings: 2

## Ingredients:

- 1 organic egg, beaten
- ½ cup Mozzarella cheese, shredded
- 2 tablespoons almond flour
- 1 tablespoon sugar-free pumpkin puree
- 1 teaspoon Erythritol
- ¼ teaspoon ground cinnamon
- 2 tablespoons walnuts, toasted and chopped

## Directions:

1. Preheat a mini waffle iron and then grease it.
2. In a bowl, place all ingredients except walnuts and beat until well combined.
3. Fold in the walnuts.
4. Place half of the mixture into preheated waffle iron and cook for about 5 minutes or until golden brown.

5. Repeat with the remaining mixture.

6. Serve warm.

## Nutrition:

Calories:148   Net   Carb:1.6g   Fat:11.8g   Saturated   Fat:2g
Carbohydrates: 3.3g Dietary Fiber: 1. Sugar: 0.8g Protein: 6.7g

# Protein Mozzarella Chaffles

Preparation time: 8 minutes

Cooking Time: 20 Minutes

Servings: 2

## Ingredients:

- ½ scoop unsweetened protein powder
- 2 large organic eggs
- ½ cup Mozzarella cheese, shredded
- 1 tablespoon Erythritol
- ¼ teaspoon organic vanilla extract

## Directions:

1. Preheat a mini waffle iron and then grease it.
2. In a medium bowl, place all ingredients and with a fork, mix until well combined.
3. Place ¼ of the mixture into preheated waffle iron and cook for about 4-5 minutes or until golden brown.
4. Repeat with the remaining mixture.
5. Serve warm.

**Nutrition:**

Calories: Net Carb:0.4g Fat:3.3g Saturated Fat:1.2g Carbohydrates: 0.4g Dietary Fiber: 0g Sugar: 0.2g Protein: 7.3g

# Chocolate Chips Peanut Butter Chaffles

Preparation time: 5 minutes

Cooking Time: 8 Minutes

Servings: 4

## Ingredients:

- 1 organic egg, beaten
- ¼ cup Mozzarella cheese, shredded
- 2 tablespoons creamy peanut butter
- 1 tablespoon almond flour
- 1 tablespoon granulated Erythritol
- 1 teaspoon organic vanilla extract
- 1 tablespoon 70% dark chocolate chips

## Directions:

1. Preheat a mini waffle iron and then grease it.
2. In a bowl, place all ingredients except chocolate chips and beat until well combined.
3. Gently, fold in the chocolate chips.

4. Place half of the mixture into preheated waffle iron and cook for about minutes or until golden brown.
5. Repeat with the remaining mixture.
6. Serve warm.

**Nutrition:**

Calories:214 Net Carb:4.1g Fat:16.8g Saturated Fat:5.4g Carbohydrates: 6.4g Dietary Fiber: 2.3g Sugar: 2.1g Protein: 8.8g

# Pumpkin Chaffles

Preparation time: 5 minutes

Cooking Time: 12 Minutes

Servings: 3

## Ingredients:

- 1 organic egg, beaten
- ½ cup Mozzarella cheese, shredded
- 1½ tablespoon homemade pumpkin puree
- ½ teaspoon Erythritol
- ½ teaspoon organic vanilla extract
- ¼ teaspoon pumpkin pie spice

## Directions:

1. Preheat a mini waffle iron and then grease it.
2. In a bowl, place all the ingredients and beat until well combined.
3. Place ¼ of the mixture into preheated waffle iron and cook for about 4-6 minutes or until golden brown.
4. Repeat with the remaining mixture.
5. Serve warm.

## Nutrition:

Calories:59 Net Carb:1.2g Fat:3.5g Saturated Fat:1.5g
Carbohydrates: 1. Dietary Fiber: 0.4g Sugar: 0.7g Protein: 4.9g

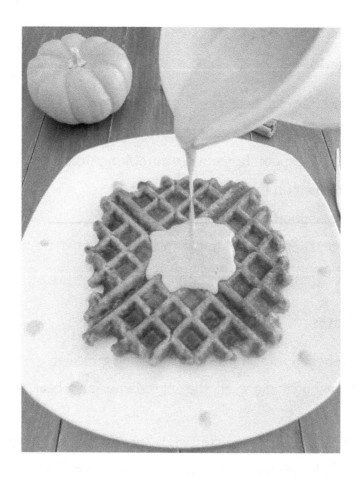

# Peanut Butter Chaffles

Preparation time: 5 minutes

Cooking Time: 8 Minutes

Servings: 2

## Ingredients:

- 1 organic egg, beaten
- ½ cup Mozzarella cheese, shredded
- 3 tablespoons granulated Erythritol
- 2 tablespoons peanut butter

## Directions:

1. Preheat a mini waffle iron and then grease it.
2. In a medium bowl, place all ingredients and with a fork, mix until well combined.
3. Place half of the mixture into preheated waffle iron and cook for about 4 minutes or until golden brown.
4. Repeat with the remaining mixture.
5. Serve warm.

**Nutrition:**

Calories:145    Net    Carb:2.    Fat:11.5g    Saturated    Fat:3.1g
Carbohydrates: 3.6g Dietary Fiber: 1g Sugar: 1.7g Protein: 8.8g

# Chocolate Chips Chaffles

Preparation time: 5 minutes

Cooking Time: 8 Minutes

Servings: 2

## Ingredients:

- 1 large organic egg
- 1 teaspoon coconut flour
- 1 teaspoon Erythritol
- ½ teaspoon organic vanilla extract
- ½ cup Mozzarella cheese, shredded finely
- 2 tablespoons 70% dark chocolate chips

## Directions:

1. Preheat a mini waffle iron and then grease it.
2. In a bowl, place the egg, coconut flour, sweetener and vanilla extract and beat until well combined.
3. Add the cheese and stir to combine.
4. Place half of the mixture into preheated waffle iron and top with half of the chocolate chips.

5. Place a little egg mixture over each chocolate chip.
6. Cook for about 3-4 minutes or until golden brown.
7. Repeat with the remaining mixture and chocolate chips.
8. Serve warm.

## Nutrition:

Calories:164 Net Carb:2. Fat:11.9g Saturated Fat:6.6g Carbohydrates: 5.4g Dietary Fiber: 2.5g Sugar: 0.3g Protein: 7.3g

# Cream Cake Chaffle

Preparation time: 8 minutes

Cooking Time: 12 Minutes

Servings: 2

**Ingredients:**

**Chaffle**

- 4 oz cream cheese, softened
- 4 eggs
- 4 tbsp coconut flour
- 1 tbsp almond flour
- 1 ½ tsp baking powder
- 1 tbsp butter, softened
- 1 tsp vanilla extract
- ½ tsp cinnamon
- 1 tbsp sweetener
- 1 tbsp shredded coconut, colored and unsweetened
- 1 tbsp walnuts, chopped

## Italian Cream Frosting

- 2 oz cream cheese, softened
- 2 tbsp butter, room temperature
- 2 tbsp sweetener
- ½ tsp vanilla

## Directions:

1. Preheat your waffle maker and add ¼ of the
2. Cook for 3 minutes and repeat the process until you have 4 chaffles.
3. Remove and set aside.
4. In the meantime, start making your frosting by mixing all the
5. Stir until you have a smooth and creamy mixture.
6. Cool, frost the cake and enjoy.

## Nutrition:

Calories per Servings: 127 Kcal ; Fats: 10 g ; Carbs: 5.5 g ; Protein: 7 g

# Almond Butter Chaffles

Preparation time: 5 minutes

Cooking Time: 10 Minutes

Servings: 2

## Ingredients:

- 1 large organic egg, beaten
- 1/3 cup Mozzarella cheese, shredded
- 1 tablespoon Erythritol
- 2 tablespoons almond butter
- 1 teaspoon organic vanilla extract

## Directions:

1. Preheat a mini waffle iron and then grease it.
2. In a medium bowl, place all ingredients and with a fork, mix until well combined.
3. Place half of the mixture into preheated waffle iron and cook for about 5 minutes or until golden brown.
4. Repeat with the remaining mixture.
5. Serve warm.

**Nutrition:**

Calories:153    Net    Carb:2g    Fat:12.3g    Saturated    Fat:2g
Carbohydrates: 3. Dietary Fiber: 1.6g Sugar: 1.2gProtein: 7.9g

# Layered Chaffles

Preparation time: 5 minutes

Cooking Time: 10 Minutes

Servings: 2

## Ingredients:

- 1 organic egg, beaten and divided
- ½ cup cheddar cheese, shredded and divided
- Pinch of salt

## Directions:

1. Preheat a mini waffle iron and then grease it.
2. Place about 1/8 cup of cheese in the bottom of the waffle iron and top with half of the beaten egg.
3. Now, place 1/8 cup of cheese on top and cook for about 4–5 minutes.
4. Repeat with the remaining cheese and egg.
5. Serve warm.

## Nutrition:

Calories 145 Net Carbs 0.5 g Total Fat 11.g Saturated Fat 6.6 g Cholesterol 112 mg Sodium 284 g Total Carbs 0.5 g Fiber 0 g Sugar 0.3 g Protein 9.8 g

# Simple Mozzarella Chaffles

Preparation time: 5 minutes

Cooking Time: 8 Minutes

Servings: 2

## Ingredients:

- ½ cup mozzarella cheese, shredded
- 1 large organic egg
- 2 tablespoons blanched almond flour
- ¼ teaspoon organic baking powder
- 2–3 drops liquid stevia

## Directions:

1. Preheat a mini waffle iron and then grease it.
2. In a medium bowl, put all ingredients and with a fork, mix until well combined. Place half of the mixture into preheated waffle iron and cook for about 3–4 minutes.
3. Repeat with the remaining mixture.
4. Serve warm.

**Nutrition:**

Calories 98 Net Carbs 1.4 g Total Fat 7.1 g Saturated Fat 1.8 g Cholesterol 97 mg Sodium 81 mg Total Carbs 2.2 g Fiber 0.8 g Sugar 0.2 g Protein 6.7 g

# Cream Mini-chaffles

Preparation time: 5 minutes

Cooking Time: 10 Minutes

Servings: 2

## Ingredients:

- 2 tsp coconut flour
- 4 tsp swerve/monk fruit
- ¼ tsp baking powder
- 1 egg
- 1 oz cream cheese
- ½ tsp vanilla extract

## Directions:

1. Turn on waffle maker to heat and oil it with cooking spray.
2. Mix swerve/monk fruit, coconut flour, and baking powder in a small mixing bowl.
3. Add cream cheese, egg, vanilla extract, and whisk until well-combined.

4. Add batter into waffle maker and cook for 3-minutes, until golden brown.

5. Serve with your favorite toppings.

## Nutrition:

Carbs: 4 g ; Fat: g ;Protein: 2 g ;Calories: 73

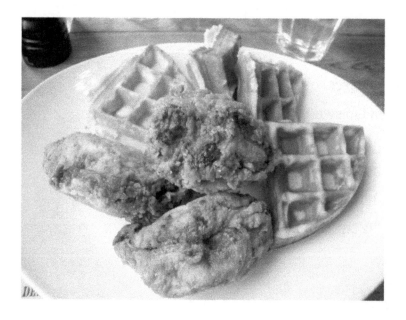

# Raspberry Chaffles

Preparation time: 5 minutes

Cooking Time: 5 Minutes

Servings: 5

## Ingredients:

- 4 Tbsp almond flour
- 4 large eggs
- 2 ⅓ cup shredded mozzarella cheese
- 1 tsp vanilla extract
- 1 Tbsp erythritol sweetener
- 1½ tsp baking powder
- ½ cup raspberries

## Directions:

1. Turn on waffle maker to heat and oil it with cooking spray.
2. Mix almond flour, sweetener, and baking powder in a bowl.

3. Add cheese, eggs, and vanilla extract, and mix until well-combined.

4. Add 1 portion of batter to waffle maker and spread it evenly. Close and cook for 3-minutes, or until golden.

5. Repeat until remaining batter is used.

6. Serve with raspberries.

## Nutrition:

Carbs: 5 g ; Fat: 11 g ;Protein: 24 g ;Calories: 300

# Lemon Chaffles

Preparation time: 5 minutes

Cooking Time: 10 Minutes

Servings: 2

## Ingredients:

- 1 organic egg, beaten
- 1 ounce cream cheese, softened
- 2 tablespoons almond flour
- 1 tablespoon fresh lemon juice
- 2 teaspoons Erythritol
- ½ teaspoon fresh lemon zest, grated
- ¼ teaspoon organic baking powder
- Pinch of salt
- ½ teaspoon powdered Erythritol

## Directions:

1. Preheat a mini waffle iron and then grease it.
2. In a bowl, place all ingredients except the powdered Erythritol and beat until well combined.

3.  Place half of the mixture into preheated waffle iron and cook for about 5 minutes or until golden brown.
4.  Repeat with the remaining mixture.
5.  Serve warm with the sprinkling of powdered Erythritol.

## Nutrition:

Calories:129 Net Carb:1.2g Fat:10.9g Saturated Fat:4.1g Carbohydrates: 2.4g Dietary Fiber: 0.8g Sugar: 0. Protein: 3.9g

# Chocolate Chip Chaffles

Preparation time: 8 minutes

Servings: 1

Cooking Time: 6 Minutes

## Ingredients:

- 1 egg
- 1 tsp coconut flour
- 1 tsp sweetener
- ½ tsp vanilla extract
- ¼ cup heavy whipping cream, for serving
- ½ cup almond milk ricotta, finely shredded
- 2 tbsp sugar-free chocolate chips

## Directions:

1. Preheat your mini waffle iron.
2. Mix the egg, coconut flour, vanilla, and sweetener. Whisk together with a fork.
3. Stir in the almond milk ricotta.

4. Pour half of the batter into the waffle iron and dot with a pinch of chocolate chips.
5. Close the waffle iron and cook for minutes.
6. Repeat with remaining batter.
7. Serve hot with the whipped cream.

**Nutrition:**

Calories per Servings: 304 Kcal ; Fats: 16 g ; Carbs: 7 g ; Protein: 3 g

# Pumpkin & Psyllium Husk Chaffles

Preparation time: 8 minutes

Cooking Time: 16 Minutes

Servings: 2

## Ingredients:

- 2 organic eggs
- ½ cup mozzarella cheese, shredded
- 1 tablespoon homemade pumpkin puree
- 2 teaspoons Erythritol
- ½ teaspoon psyllium husk powder
- 1/3 teaspoon ground cinnamon
- Pinch of salt
- ½ teaspoon organic vanilla extract

## Directions:

1. Preheat a mini waffle iron and then grease it.
2. In a bowl, place all ingredients and beat until well combined.

3.  Place ¼ of the mixture into preheated waffle iron and cook for about 4 minutes or until golden brown.
4.  Repeat with the remaining mixture.
5.  Serve warm.


## Nutrition:

Calories:4et    Carb:0.6g    Fat:2.8g    Saturated    Fat:1.1g Carbohydrates: 0.8g Dietary Fiber: 0.2g Sugar: 0.4g Protein: 3.9g

# Blackberry Chaffles

Preparation time: 5 minutes

Cooking Time: 8 Minutes

Servings: 2

## Ingredients:

- 1 organic egg, beaten
- 1/3 cup Mozzarella cheese, shredded
- 1 teaspoon cream cheese, softened
- 1 teaspoon coconut flour
- ¼ teaspoon organic baking powder
- ¾ teaspoon powdered Erythritol
- ¼ teaspoon ground cinnamon
- ¼ teaspoon organic vanilla extract
- Pinch of salt
- 1 tablespoon fresh blackberries

## Directions:

1. Preheat a mini waffle iron and then grease it.

2. In a bowl, place all ingredients except for blackberries and beat until well combined.

3. Fold in the blackberries.

4. Place half of the mixture into preheated waffle iron and cook for about minutes or until golden brown.

5. Repeat with the remaining mixture.

6. Serve warm.

## Nutrition:

Calories:121   Net   Carb:2.   Fat:7.5g   Saturated   Fat:3.3g Carbohydrates: 4.5g Dietary Fiber: 1.8g Sugar: 0.9gProtein: 8.9g

# Pumpkin Cream Cheese Chaffles

Preparation time: 5 minutes

Cooking Time: 10 Minutes

Servings: 2

## Ingredients:

- 1 organic egg, beaten
- ½ cup Mozzarella cheese, shredded
- 1½ tablespoon sugar-free pumpkin puree
- 2 teaspoons heavy cream
- 1 teaspoon cream cheese, softened
- 1 tablespoon almond flour
- 1 tablespoon Erythritol
- ½ teaspoon pumpkin pie spice
- ½ teaspoon organic baking powder
- 1 teaspoon organic vanilla extract

## Directions:

1. Preheat a mini waffle iron and then grease it.

2. In a medium bowl, place all ingredients and with a fork, mix until well combined.

3. Place half of the mixture into preheated waffle iron and cook for about 5 minutes or until golden brown.

4. Repeat with the remaining mixture.

5. Serve warm.

## Nutrition:

Calories:110 Net Carb:2.5g Fat:4.3g Saturated Fat:1g Carbohydrates: 3.3g Dietary Fiber: 0.8g Sugar: 1g Protein: 5.2g

# Cinnamon Pecan Chaffles

Preparation time: 5 minutes

Servings: 1

Cooking Time: 40 Minutes

## Ingredients:

- 1 Tbsp butter
- 1 egg
- ½ tsp vanilla
- 2 Tbsp almond flour
- 1 Tbsp coconut flour
- ⅛ tsp baking powder
- 1 Tbsp monk fruit

## For the crumble:

- ½ tsp cinnamon
- 1 Tbsp melted butter
- 1 tsp monk fruit
- 1 Tbsp chopped pecans

## Directions:

1. Turn on waffle maker to heat and oil it with cooking spray.
2. Melt butter in a bowl, then mix in the egg and vanilla.
3. Mix in remaining chaffle ingredients.
4. Combine crumble ingredients in a separate bowl.
5. Pour half of the chaffle mix into waffle maker. Top with half of crumble mixture.
6. Cook for 5 minutes, or until done.
7. Repeat with the other half of the batter.

## Nutrition:

Carbs: g ; Fat: 35 g ; Protein: 10 g ; Calories: 391

# Chaffle Glazed with Raspberry

Preparation time: 5 minutes

Servings: 1

Cooking Time: 5 Minutes

**Ingredients:**

**Donut Chaffle Ingredients:**

- 1 egg
- ¼ cup mozzarella cheese, shredded
- 2 tsp cream cheese, softened
- 1 tsp sweetener
- 1tsp almond flour
- ½ tsp baking powder
- 20 drops glazed donut flavoring

**Raspberry Jelly Filling:**

- ¼ cup raspberries
- 1 tsp chia seeds
- 1 tsp confectioners' sweetener

## Donut Glaze:

- 1 tsp powdered sweetener
- Heavy whipping cream

## Directions:

1. Spray your waffle maker with cooking oil and add the butter mixture into the waffle maker.
2. Cook for 3 minutes and set aside.

## Raspberry Jelly Filling:

3. Mix all the
4. Place in a pot and heat on medium.
5. Gently mash the raspberries and set aside to cool.

## Donut Glaze:

6. Stir together the

## Assembling:

7. Lay your chaffles on a plate and add the fillings mixture between the layers.
8. Drizzle the glaze on top and enjoy.

## Nutrition:

Calories per Servings: 188 Kcal ; Fats: 23 g ; Carbs: 12 g ; Protein: 17 g

# Biscuit Keto Chaffles

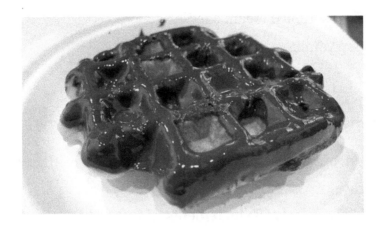

Preparation time: 5 minutes

Cooking Time: 5 Minutes

Servings: 2


## Ingredients:

- 1 egg
- 1½ Tbsp unsweetened cocoa
- 2 Tbsp lakanto monk fruit, or choice of sweetener
- 1 Tbsp heavy cream
- 1 tsp coconut flour
- ½ tsp baking powder
- ½ tsp vanilla

## For the cheese cream:

- 1 Tbsp lakanto powdered sweetener
- 2 Tbsp softened cream cheese
- ¼ tsp vanilla

## Directions:

1. Turn on waffle maker to heat and oil it with cooking spray.
2. Combine all chaffle ingredients in a small bowl.
3. Pour one half of the chaffle mixture into waffle maker. Cook for 5 minutes.
4. Remove and repeat with the second half if the mixture. Let chaffles sit for 2-3 to crisp up.
5. Combine all cream ingredients and spread on chaffle when they have cooled to room temperature.

## Nutrition:

Carbs: 3 g ; Fat: 4 g ;Protein: 7 g ;Calories:

# Cinnamon Sugar Chaffles

Preparation time: 5 minutes

Cooking Time: 12 Minutes

Servings: 2

## Ingredients:

- 2 eggs
- 1 cup Mozzarella cheese, shredded
- 2 tbsp blanched almond flour
- ½ tbsp butter, melted
- 2 tbsp Erythritol
- ½ tsp cinnamon
- ½ tsp vanilla extract
- ½ tsp psyllium husk powder, optional
- ¼ tsp baking powder, optional
- 1 tbsp melted butter, for topping
- ¼ cup Erythritol, for topping
- ¾ tsp cinnamon, for topping

## Directions:

1. Pour enough batter into the waffle maker and cook for 4 minutes.
2. Once the cooked, carefully remove the chaffle and set aside.
3. Repeat with the remaining batter the same steps.
4. Stir together the cinnamon and erythritol.
5. Finish by brushing your chaffles with the melted butter and then sprinkle with cinnamon sugar.

## Nutrition:

Calories 108 Kcal ; Fats: 16 g ; Carbs: 4 g ; Protein: 11 g

# Cream Cheese Chaffles

Preparation time: 5 minutes

Cooking Time: 8 Minutes

Servings: 2

## Ingredients:

- 2 teaspoons coconut flour
- 3 teaspoons Erythritol
- ¼ teaspoon organic baking powder
- 1 organic egg, beaten
- 1 ounce cream cheese, softened
- ½ teaspoon organic vanilla extract

## Directions:

1. Preheat a mini waffle iron and then grease it.
2. In a bowl, place flour, Erythritol and baking powder and mix well.
3. Add the egg, cream cheese and vanilla extract and beat until well combined.

4. Place half of the mixture into preheated waffle iron and cook for about 3-minutes or until golden brown.
5. Repeat with the remaining mixture.
6. Serve warm.

## Nutrition:

Calories:95 Net Carb: 1.6g Fat: 4g Saturated Fat: 4g Carbohydrates: 2.6g Dietary Fiber: 1g Sugar: 0.3g Protein: 4.2g

# Mozzarella & Butter Chaffles

Preparation time: 5 minutes

Cooking Time: 8 Minutes

Servings: 2

## Ingredients:

- 1 large organic egg, beaten
- ¾ cup Mozzarella cheese, shredded
- ½ tablespoon unsalted butter, melted
- 2 tablespoons blanched almond flour
- 2 tablespoons Erythritol
- ½ teaspoon ground cinnamon
- ½ teaspoon Psyllium husk powder
- ¼ teaspoon organic baking powder
- ½ teaspoon organic vanilla extract

## Directions:

1. Preheat a waffle iron and then grease it.
2. In a medium bowl, place all ingredients and with a fork, mix until well combined.

3. Place half of the mixture into preheated waffle iron and cook for about 5 minutes or until golden brown.
4. Repeat with the remaining mixture.
5. Serve warm.

## Nutrition:

Calories:140    Net    Carb:1.9g    Fat:10.    Saturated    Fat:4g Carbohydrates: 3g Dietary Fiber: 1.1g Sugar: 0.3g Protein: 7.8g

# Pumpkin Pecan Chaffles

Preparation time: 5 minutes

Cooking Time: 10 Minutes

Servings: 2

## Ingredients:

- 1 egg
- ½ cup mozzarella cheese grated
- 1 Tbsp pumpkin puree
- ½ tsp pumpkin spice
- 1 tsp erythritol low carb sweetener
- 2 Tbsp almond flour
- 2 Tbsp pecans, toasted chopped
- 1 cup heavy whipped cream
- ¼ cup low carb caramel sauce

## Directions:

1. Turn on waffle maker to heat and oil it with cooking spray.
2. In a bowl, beat egg.

3. Mix in mozzarella, pumpkin, flour, pumpkin spice, and erythritol.

4. Stir in pecan pieces.

5. Spoon one half of the batter into waffle maker and spread evenly.

6. Close and cook for 5 minutes.

7. Remove cooked waffles to a plate.

8. Repeat with remaining batter.

9. Serve with pecans, whipped cream, and low carb caramel sauce.

**Nutrition:**

Carbs: 4 g ; Fat: 17 g ; Protein: 11 g ; Calories: 210

# Chocolate Cream Chaffles

Preparation time: 5 minutes

Cooking Time: 10 Minutes

Servings: 2

## Ingredients:

- 1 organic egg
- 1½ tablespoons cacao powder
- 2 tablespoons Erythritol
- 1 tablespoon heavy cream
- 1 teaspoon coconut flour
- ½ teaspoon organic baking powder
- ½ teaspoon organic vanilla extract
- ½ teaspoon powdered Erythritol

## Directions:

1. Preheat a mini waffle iron and then grease it.
2. In a bowl, place all ingredients except the powdered Erythritol and beat until well combined.

3. Place half of the mixture into preheated waffle iron and cook for about 5 minutes or until golden brown.
4. Repeat with the remaining mixture.
5. Serve warm with the sprinkling of powdered Erythritol.

**Nutrition:**

Calories: 7et Carb: 2.1g Fat: 5.9g Saturated Fat: 3g Carbohydrates:

3.8g Dietary Fiber: 1.7g Sugar: 0.3g Protein: 3.8g

# Blueberry Cinnamon Chaffles

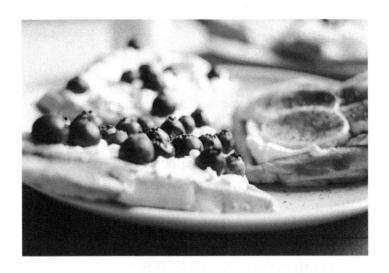

Preparation time: 5 minutes

Servings: 3

Cooking Time: 10 Minutes


**Ingredients:**

- 1 cup shredded mozzarella cheese
- 3 Tbsp almond flour
- 2 eggs
- 2 tsp Swerve or granulated sweetener of choice
- 1 tsp cinnamon
- ½ tsp baking powder

- ½ cup fresh blueberries
- ½ tsp of powdered Swerve

## Directions:

1. Turn on waffle maker to heat and oil it with cooking spray.
2. Mix eggs, flour, mozzarella, cinnamon, vanilla extract, sweetener, and baking powder in a bowl until well combined.
3. Add in blueberries.
4. Pour ¼ batter into each waffle mold.
5. Close and cook for 8 minutes.
6. If it's crispy and the waffle maker opens without pulling the chaffles apart, the chaffle is ready. If not, close and cook for 1-2 minutes more.
7. Serve with favorite topping and more blueberries.

## Nutrition:

Carbs: 9 g ; Fat: 12 g ; Protein: 13 g ; Calories: 193

# Gingerbread Chaffle

Preparation time: 5 minutes

Cooking Time: 5 Minutes

Servings: 2

## Ingredients:

- ½ cup mozzarella cheese grated
- 1 medium egg
- ½ tsp baking powder
- 1 tsp erythritol powdered
- ½ tsp ground ginger
- ¼ tsp ground nutmeg
- ½ tsp ground cinnamon
- ⅛ tsp ground cloves
- 2 Tbsp almond flour
- 1 cup heavy whipped cream
- ¼ cup keto-friendly maple syrup

## Directions:

1. Turn on waffle maker to heat and oil it with cooking spray.
2. Beat egg in a bowl.
3. Add flour, mozzarella, spices, baking powder, and erythritol. Mix well.
4. Spoon one half of the batter into waffle maker and spread out evenly.
5. Close and cook for minutes.
6. Remove cooked chaffle and repeat with remaining batter.
7. Serve with whipped cream and maple syrup.


## Nutrition:

Carbs: 5 g ; Fat: 15 g ; Protein: 12 g ; Calories: 103

# Chocolate Whipping Cream Chaffles

Preparation time: 5 minutes

Cooking Time: 8 Minutes

Servings: 2

## Ingredients:

- 1 tablespoon almond flour
- 2 tablespoons cacao powder
- 2 tablespoons granulated Erythritol
- ¼ teaspoon organic baking powder
- 1 organic egg
- 1 tablespoon heavy whipping cream
- ¼ teaspoon organic vanilla extract
- 1/8 teaspoon organic almond extract

## Directions:

1. Preheat a mini waffle iron and then grease it.
2. In a bowl, place all ingredients and beat until well combined.

3. Place half of the mixture into preheated waffle iron and cook for about 4 minutes or until golden brown.
4. Repeat with the remaining mixture.
5. Serve warm.

**Nutrition**:

Calories:94 Net Carb:2g Fat:7.9g Saturated Fat:3.2g Carbohydrates: 3.9g Dietary Fiber: 1.9g Sugar: 0.4g Protein: 3.9g

# Almond Flour Chaffles

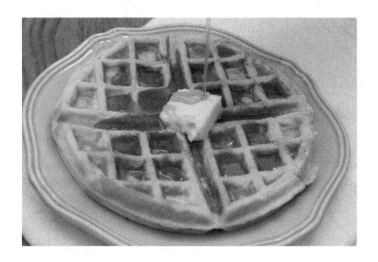

Preparation time: 5 minutes

Cooking Time: 20 Minutes

Servings: 2

## Ingredients:

- 1 large egg
- 1 Tbsp blanched almond flour
- ¼ tsp baking powder
- ½ cup shredded mozzarella cheese

## Directions:

1. Whisk egg, almond flour, and baking powder together.
2. Stir in mozzarella and set batter aside.
3. Turn on waffle maker to heat and oil it with cooking spray.
4. Pour half of the batter onto waffle maker and spread it evenly with a spoon.
5. Cook for 3 minutes, or until it reaches desired doneness.
6. Transfer to a plate and repeat with remaining batter.
7. Let chaffles cool for 2-3 minutes to crisp up.

## Nutrition:

Carbs: 2 g ; Fat: 13 g ;Protein: 10 g ; Calories: 131

# Strawberry cake Chaffles

Preparation time: 5 minutes

Servings: 1

Cooking Time: 25 Minutes

**Ingredients:**

**For the batter:**

- 1 egg
- ¼ cup mozzarella cheese
- 1 Tbsp cream cheese
- ¼ tsp baking powder
- 2 strawberries, sliced
- 1 tsp strawberry extract

**For the glaze:**

- 1 Tbsp cream cheese
- ¼ tsp strawberry extract
- 1 Tbsp monk fruit confectioners blend

## For the whipped cream:

- 1 cup heavy whipping cream
- 1 tsp vanilla
- 1 Tbsp monk fruit

## Directions:

1. Turn on waffle maker to heat and oil it with cooking spray.
2. Beat egg in a small bowl.
3. Add remaining batter components.
4. Divide the mixture in half.
5. Cook one half of the batter in a waffle maker for 4 minutes, or until golden brown.Repeat with remaining batter
6. Mix all glaze ingredients and spread over each warm chaffle.
7. Mix all whipped cream ingredients and whip until it starts to form peaks.
8. Top each waffle with whipped cream and strawberries.

## Nutrition:

Carbs: 5 g ; Fat: 14 g ; Protein: 12 g ; Calories: 218

# Cream Cheese & Butter Chaffles

Preparation time: 8 minutes

Cooking Time: 16 Minutes

Servings: 2

## Ingredients:

- 2 tablespoons butter, melted and cooled
- 2 large organic eggs
- 2 ounces cream cheese, softened
- ¼ cup powdered Erythritol
- 1½ teaspoons organic vanilla extract
- Pinch of salt
- ¼ cup almond flour
- 2 tablespoons coconut flour
- 1 teaspoon organic baking powder

## Directions:

1. Preheat a mini waffle iron and then grease it.
2. In a bowl, place the butter and eggs and beat until creamy.

3. Add the cream cheese, Erythritol, vanilla extract and salt and beat until well combined.

4. Add the flours and baking powder and beat until well combined.

5. Place ¼ of the mixture into preheated waffle iron and cook for about 4 minutes or until golden brown.

6. Repeat with the remaining mixture.

7. Serve warm.

**Nutrition:**

Calories:202 Net Carb:2. Fat:17.3g Saturated Fat:8g Carbohydrates: 5.1g Dietary Fiber: 2.3g Sugar: 0.7g Protein: 4.8g

# Chocolate Cherry Chaffles

Preparation time: 5 minutes

Servings: 1

Cooking Time: 5 Minutes

## Ingredients:

- 1 Tbsp almond flour
- 1 Tbsp cocoa powder
- 1 Tbsp sugar free sweetener
- ½ tsp baking powder
- 1 whole egg
- ½ cup mozzarella cheese shredded
- 2 Tbsp heavy whipping cream whipped
- 2 Tbsp sugar free cherry pie filling
- 1 Tbsp chocolate chips

## Directions:

1. Turn on waffle maker to heat and oil it with cooking spray.
2. Mix all dry components in a bowl.
3. Add egg and mix well.

4. Add cheese and stir again.

5. Spoon batter into waffle maker and close.

6. Cook for 5 minutes, until done.

7. Top with whipping cream, cherries, and chocolate chips.

## Nutrition:

Carbs: 6 g ; Fat: 1 g ; Protein: 1 g ; Calories: 130

# Coconut & Walnut Chaffles

Preparation time: 5 minutes

Servings: 8

Cooking Time: 24 Minutes

## Ingredients:

- 4 organic eggs, beaten
- 4 ounces cream cheese, softened
- 1 tablespoon butter, melted
- 4 tablespoons coconut flour
- 1 tablespoon almond flour
- 2 tablespoons Erythritol
- 1½ teaspoons organic baking powder
- 1 teaspoon organic vanilla extract
- ½ teaspoon ground cinnamon
- 1 tablespoon unsweetened coconut, shredded
- 1 tablespoon walnuts, chopped

## Directions:

1. Preheat a mini waffle iron and then grease it.
2. In a blender, place all ingredients and pulse until creamy and smooth.
3. Divide the mixture into 8 portions.
4. Place 1 portion of the mixture into preheated waffle iron and cook for about 2-3 minutes or until golden brown.
5. Repeat with the remaining mixture.
6. Serve warm.

## Nutrition:

Calories:125   Net   Carb:2.2g   Fat:10.2g   Saturated   Fat:5.2g Carbohydrates: 4g Dietary Fiber: 1.8g Sugar: 0.4g Protein: 4.6g

# Chocolate Chaffles

Preparation time: 5 minutes

Cooking Time: 10 Minutes

Servings: 2

## Ingredients:

- ¾ cup shredded mozzarella
- 1 large egg
- 2 Tbsp almond flour
- 2 Tbsp allulose
- ½ Tbsp melted butter
- 1½ Tbsp cocoa powder
- ½ tsp vanilla extract
- ½ tsp psyllium husk powder
- ¼ tsp baking powder

## Directions:

1. Turn on waffle maker to heat and oil it with cooking spray.
2. Mix all ingredients in a small bowl.

3. Pour ¼ cup batter into a 4-inch waffle maker.
4. Cook for 2-3 minutes, or until crispy.
5. Transfer chaffle to a plate and set aside.
6. Repeat with remaining batter.

**Nutrition:**

Carbs: 6 g ; Fat: 24 g ; Protein: 15 g ; Calories: 296

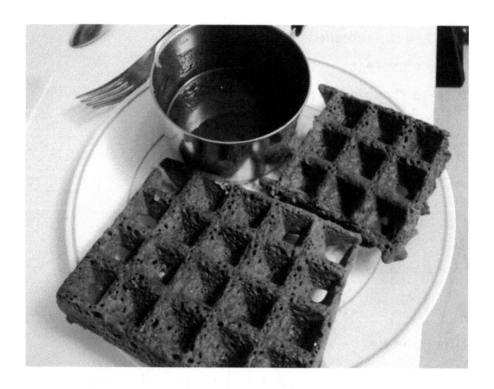

# Chocolate Chips & Whipping Cream Chaffles

Preparation time: 5 minutes

Cooking Time: 8 Minutes

Servings: 2

## Ingredients:

- 1 organic egg
- 1 tablespoon heavy whipping cream
- ½ teaspoon coconut flour
- 1¾ teaspoons monk fruit sweetener
- ¼ teaspoon organic baking powder
- Pinch of salt
- 1 tablespoon 70% dark chocolate chips

## Directions:

1. Preheat a mini waffle iron and then grease it.
2. In a bowl, place all ingredients except for chocolate chips and beat until well combined.

3. Fold in the blackberries.

4. Place half of the mixture into preheated waffle iron and top with half of the chocolate chips.

5. Cook for about 3-4 minutes or until golden brown.

6. Repeat with the remaining mixture and chocolate chips.

7. Serve warm.

## Nutrition:

Calories: 110 Net Carb: 1. Fat: 9g Saturated Fat: 5g Carbohydrates:3.1g Dietary Fiber: 1.3g Sugar: 0.2g Protein: 4g

# Spiced Pumpkin Chaffles

Preparation time: 5 minutes

Cooking Time: 8 Minutes

Servings: 2

## Ingredients:

- 1 organic egg, beaten
- ½ cup Mozzarella cheese, shredded
- 1 tablespoon sugar-free canned solid pumpkin
- ¼ teaspoon ground cinnamon
- Pinch of ground cloves
- Pinch of ground nutmeg
- Pinch of ground ginger

## Directions:

1. Preheat a mini waffle iron and then grease it.
2. In a medium bowl, place all ingredients and with a fork, mix until well combined.
3. Place half of the mixture into preheated waffle iron and cook for about 4 minutes or until golden brown.

4. Repeat with the remaining mixture.

5. Serve warm.

## Nutrition:

Calories:5et     Carb:1g     Fat:3.5g     Saturated     Fat:1.5g
Carbohydrates:1.4g Dietary Fiber: 0.4g Sugar: 0.5g Protein: 4.9g

# Vanilla Chaffle

Preparation time: 5 minutes

Cooking Time: 8 Minutes

Servings: 4

## Ingredients:

- 2 tbsp butter, softened
- 2 oz cream cheese, softened
- 2 eggs
- ¼ cup almond flour
- 2 tbsp coconut flour
- 1 tsp baking powder
- 1 tsp vanilla extract
- ¼ cup confectioners
- Pinch of pink salt

## Directions:

1. Preheat the waffle maker and spray with non-stick cooking spray.
2. Melt the butter and set aside for a minute to cool.

3. Add the eggs into the melted butter and whisk until creamy.

4. Pour in the sweetener, vanilla, extract, and salt. Blend properly.

5. Next add the coconut flour, almond flour, and baking powder. Mix well.

6. Pour into the waffle maker and cook for 4 minutes.

7. Repeat the process with the remaining batter.

8. Remove and set aside to cool.

9. Enjoy.

**Nutrition:**

Calories per Preparation time: 5 minutes 02 Kcal ; Fats: 27 g Carbs: 9 g ; Protein: 23 g

# Banana Nut Chaffle

Preparation time: 5 minutes

Servings: 1

Cooking Time: 10 Minutes

## Ingredients:

- 1 egg
- 1 Tbsp cream cheese, softened and room temp
- 1 Tbsp sugar-free cheesecake pudding
- ½ cup mozzarella cheese
- 1 Tbsp monk fruit confectioners' sweetener
- ¼ tsp vanilla extract
- ¼ tsp banana extract
- toppings of choice

## Directions:

1. Turn on waffle maker to heat and oil it with cooking spray.
2. Beat egg in a small bowl.

3. Add remaining ingredients and mix until well incorporated.
4. Add one half of the batter to waffle maker and cook for minutes, until golden brown.
5. Remove chaffle and add the other half of the batter.
6. Top with your optional toppings and serve warm!

## Nutrition:

Carbs: 2 g ; Fat: g ; Protein: 8 g ; Calories: 119

# Chocolaty Chips Pumpkin Chaffles

Preparation time: 5 minutes

Servings: 3

Cooking Time: 12 Minutes

## Ingredients:

- 1 organic egg
- 4 teaspoons homemade pumpkin puree
- ½ cup Mozzarella cheese, shredded
- 1 tablespoon almond flour
- 2 tablespoons granulated Erythritol
- ¼ teaspoon pumpkin pie spice
- 4 teaspoons 70% dark chocolate chips

## Directions:

1. In a bowl, place the egg and pumpkin puree and mix well.
2. Add the remaining ingredients except for chocolate chips and mix until well combined.

3. Gently, fold in the chocolate chips and lemon zest.
4. Place 1/3 of the mixture into preheated waffle iron and cook for about minutes or until golden brown.
5. Repeat with the remaining mixture.
6. Serve warm.

## Nutrition:

Calories:9et    Carb:1.9g    Fat:7.1g    Saturated    Fat:3.3g Carbohydrates: 1.4g Dietary Fiber: 2.6g Sugar: 0.4g Protein: 4.2g

# Whipping Cream Pumpkin Chaffles

Preparation time: 8 minutes

Cooking Time: 12 Minutes

Servings: 2

## Ingredients:

- 2 organic eggs
- 2 tablespoons homemade pumpkin puree
- 2 tablespoons heavy whipping cream
- 1 tablespoon coconut flour
- 1 tablespoon Erythritol
- 1 teaspoon pumpkin pie spice
- ½ teaspoon organic baking powder
- ½ teaspoon organic vanilla extract
- Pinch of salt
- ½ cup Mozzarella cheese, shredded

## Directions:

1. Preheat a mini waffle iron and then grease it.
2. In a bowl, place all the ingredients except Mozzarella cheese and beat until well combined.
3. Add the Mozzarella cheese and stir to combine.
4. Place half of the mixture into preheated waffle iron and cook for about 6 minutes or until golden brown.
5. Repeat with the remaining mixture.
6. Serve warm.

## Nutrition:

Calories:81 Net Carb2.1g Fat:5.9g Saturated Fat:3g Carbohydrates: 3.1g Dietary Fiber: 1g Sugar: 0.5g Protein: 4.3g

# Chocolate Vanilla Chaffles

Preparation time: 5 minutes

Cooking Time: 5 Minutes

Servings: 2

## Ingredients:

- ½ cup shredded mozzarella cheese
- 1 egg
- 1 Tbsp granulated sweetener
- 1 tsp vanilla extract
- 1 Tbsp sugar-free chocolate chips
- 2 Tbsp almond meal/flour

## Directions:

1. Turn on waffle maker to heat and oil it with cooking spray.
2. Mix all components in a bowl until combined.
3. Pour half of the batter into waffle maker.
4. Cook for 2-minutes, then remove and repeat with remaining batter.

5.  Top with more chips and favorite toppings.

## Nutrition:

Carbs: 23 g ; Fat: 3 g ; Protein: 4 g ; Calories: 134

# Churro Waffles

Preparation time: 5 minutes

Servings: 1

Cooking Time: 10 Minutes

## Ingredients:

- 1 tbsp coconut cream
- 1 egg
- 6 tbsp almond flour
- ¼ tsp xanthan gum
- ½ tsp cinnamon
- 2 tbsp keto brown sugar

## Coating:

- 2 tbsp butter, melt
- 1 tbsp keto brown sugar
- Warm up your waffle maker.

## Directions:

1. Pour half of the batter to the waffle pan and cook for 5 minutes.
2. Carefully remove the cooked waffle and repeat the steps with the remaining batter.
3. Allow the chaffles to cool and spread with the melted butter and top with the brown sugar.
4. Enjoy.

## Nutrition:

Calories per Servings: 178 Kcal  ;  Fats: 15.7 g  ;  Carbs: 3.9 g ; Protein: 2 g

# Chocolate Chips Lemon Chaffles

Preparation time: 8 minutes

Cooking Time: 8 Minutes

Servings: 2

## Ingredients:

- 2 organic eggs
- ½ cup Mozzarella cheese, shredded
- ¾ teaspoon organic lemon extract
- ½ teaspoon organic vanilla extract
- 2 teaspoons Erythritol
- ½ teaspoon psyllium husk powder
- Pinch of salt
- 1 tablespoon 70% dark chocolate chips
- ¼ teaspoon lemon zest, grated finely

## Directions:

1. Preheat a mini waffle iron and then grease it.
2. In a bowl, place all ingredients except chocolate chips and lemon zest and beat until well combined.

3. Gently, fold in the chocolate chips and lemon zest.
4. Place ¼ of the mixture into preheated waffle iron and cook for about minutes or until golden brown.
5. Repeat with the remaining mixture.
6. Serve warm.

## Nutrition:

Calories: Net Carb: 1g Fat: 4.8g Saturated Fat: 2.3g Carbohydrates:1.5g Dietary Fiber: 0.5g Sugar: 0.3g Protein: 4.3g

# Mocha Chaffles

Servings: 3

Cooking Time: 9 Minutes

## Ingredients:

- 1 organic egg, beaten
- 1 tablespoon cacao powder
- 1 tablespoon Erythritol
- ¼ teaspoon organic baking powder
- 2 tablespoons cream cheese, softened
- 1 tablespoon mayonnaise
- ¼ teaspoon instant coffee powder
- Pinch of salt
- 1 teaspoon organic vanilla extract

## Directions:

1. Preheat a mini waffle iron and then grease it.
2. In a medium bowl, place all ingredients and with a fork, mix until well combined.

3. Place 1/of the mixture into preheated waffle iron and cook for about 2½-3 minutes or until golden brown.
4. Repeat with the remaining mixture.
5. Serve warm.

**Nutrition:**

Calories: 83 Net Carb: 1g Fat: 7.5g Saturated Fat: 4. Carbohydrates: 1.5g Dietary Fiber: 0.5g Sugar: 0.3g Protein: 2.7g

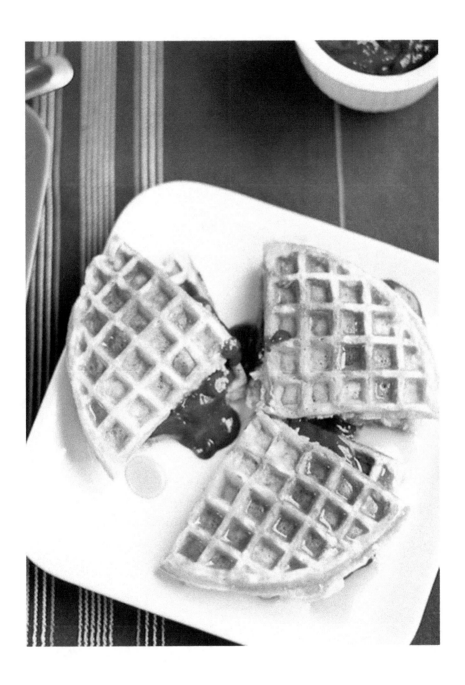

Lightning Source UK Ltd.
Milton Keynes UK
UKHW020214080521
383350UK00003B/281